HOW TO START MEAL PLANNING

MEAL PLANNING STRATEGIES FOR ALL

AHMED .R

Contents

CHAPTER ONE

INTRODUCTION

Meal planning is a smart way to arrange meals for your family or yourself ahead of time. It has several advantages, including stress relief, time savings, and the encouragement of better eating habits. Meal preparation can be a huge help, regardless of your situation you might be a working professional, a parent wanting to manage a family, or someone trying to save costs. However, where do you even begin?

Meal planning doesn't have to be difficult to begin with. You may start streamlining your meal preparation process and reap the rewards of more economical and productive eating habits with a few easy actions and techniques.

We'll go over the essential procedures in this guide to get you started with meal planning. You'll discover how to take charge of your food choices, saving time and money along the way, from goal-setting and meal planning to smart shopping and advance meal preparation. Regardless of your level of experience in the kitchen, this guide will teach you the skills and methods necessary to turn meal preparation into a pleasurable and easy part of your daily routine.

The act of planning and preparing meals ahead of time, usually for a week or other specified duration, is known as meal planning. It entails planning meals, making a shopping list, buying ingredients, and frequently cooking some or all of the meals in advance. There are many advantages to meal planning that can improve different facets of your life:

Saves Time: You may cut down on the amount of time you spend determining what to eat every day and making several trips to the grocery store by organizing your meals in advance. Meal preparation becomes more effective when you have a strategy in place, which frees up your time to cook during hectic workdays.

Lessens tension: Making meal plans helps to remove the uncertainty and tension that come with making decisions at meals. Preparing your meals ahead of time can help reduce last-minute rushing and give you a more composed and organized attitude when it comes to mealtimes.

Encourages Healthier Eating Habits: By allowing you to make more deliberate food selections, meal planning helps you maintain a balanced and nutrient-dense diet. You may enhance your general health and well-being by including a range of fruits, vegetables, lean proteins, and healthy grains in your meals.

Reduces Food Waste: Making a meal plan in advance allows you to buy only what you need and make efficient use of your ingredients. This promotes a more ecologically conscious and sustainable way of living by lowering the risk of food spoiling and minimizing food waste.

Saves Money: By minimizing impulsive purchases, cutting back on eating out, and making the most of ingredients, meal planning can result in significant cost savings. You may eat healthily and happily at home while reducing your grocery expenditure by planning your shopping and buying in bulk.

Promotes Variety: Arranging your meals ahead of time enables you to include a wide variety of foods and flavors in your diet. This guarantees that you experience a range of tastes and textures throughout the week and promotes culinary creativity. It also keeps mealtimes from becoming monotonous.

Supports Weight Management Objectives: Meal planning can be a useful tool for people who want to control their weight. Meal planning can help with weight loss or maintenance by regulating portion sizes, selecting nutrient-dense foods, and keeping an eye on calorie consumption.

Enhances Time Management: By planning meals ahead of time, you can better manage your time by allocating it to chores related to preparation. This guarantees that you have wholesome meals available when you need them and lets you manage your culinary duties with other obligations.

All things considered, meal planning is a useful and effective way to eat healthily while reducing stress, expense, and time spent cooking. Meal planning can help you reach your goals and reap the benefits of more ordered and attentive eating habits, whether your objectives are to lose weight, cut down on food waste, or simplify your daily routine.

Meal planning is essential for encouraging healthier eating habits and saving time and money.

To promote healthier eating habits and save time and money, meal planning is essential. Here are the reasons it matters in each of these areas:

Conserving Time:

Reduces Decision Fatigue: By eliminating the need to choose what to eat every day, meal planning helps people save time and mental energy.

Simplifies Meal Preparation: By planning ahead, you can cut down on cooking time during hectic workdays by preparing items ahead of time.

Reduces the Number of excursions to the Grocery Store: Making a detailed shopping list in advance of meals helps you cut down on the number of excursions to the store and save time.

Conserving Cash:

Meal planning lets you buy only what you need, which reduces food waste and helps you spend less on groceries.

Predefined lists help you avoid impulsive purchases, which will help you stick to your spending plan and save money.

Optimizes Ingredient Use: Making a meal plan helps you make the most use of your ingredients and minimizes the need for extra supermarket shopping.

Encouraging Better Eating Practices:

Promotes Balanced Nutrition: By include a range of fruits, vegetables, lean meats, and whole grains in your diet, meal planning helps you to achieve balanced nutrition.

Reducing Dependency on Processed and Unhealthy Convenience Foods: Cooking at home gives you more control over the ingredients you use.

Facilitates Portion Control: Meals that are planned increase your chances of controlling portion sizes, which helps you avoid overindulging and encourage better eating practices.

Enhances Awareness of Food Choices: Making meal plans promotes mindful eating and raises awareness of food options, which helps you make more thoughtful eating decisions.

Meal planning is an excellent way to promote healthier eating habits and save time and money. You can simplify your cooking process, stay within your budget, and make sure you're eating wholesome, filling meals on a regular basis by

Evaluating your individual requirements and preferences is a crucial first step in meal planning. Here's how to approach it:

Take into Account Dietary Restrictions and Preferences: Make a list of all the food allergies, dietary restrictions, and preferences that you and your family members may have. This could involve avoiding gluten, following a vegetarian or vegan diet, or having particular food allergies. Make sure your food plans take these requirements and inclinations into account.

Analyze Time Restraints: Look at your calendar and figure out how much time you have each week to prepare meals. In order to save time throughout the week when you have a hectic schedule, give priority to quick and simple recipes or schedule bulk cooking and meal prep for the weekends.

Evaluate Your Cooking Ability: Take into account your degree of comfort and expertise in the kitchen. Start with basic recipes if you're new to cooking or have little expertise in the kitchen, and as you develop confidence, work your way up to more complicated dishes.

Establish Health Objectives: List any objectives you have for your health, such as reducing weight, boosting your energy, or enhancing your general wellbeing. Make use of meal planning as a tool to help you achieve these objectives by making sure your plan includes wholesome, well-balanced meals.

Take Stock of Your Kitchen Equipment: Examine the cookware, appliances, pots, and pans that you currently have on hand. Make a list of any necessary kitchen appliances, such a food processor, blender, or slow cooker, that you might need to purchase.

Think About Family Preferences: When organizing a family's dinner, consider the inclinations and preferences of each family member. Engage them in the process of meal planning by getting their feedback on their favorite dishes or desired ingredient lists.

CHAPTER TWO

Analyze Financial Restraints: Establish your grocery budget and consider how meal planning can help you stick to it. To optimize savings, take into account inexpensive ingredients, purchasing in bulk, and reducing food waste.

Examine Your existing Eating Practices: Examine your existing eating practices and note any areas where you'd like to improve. This can entail eating more vegetables, cutting out on processed foods, or adding more home-cooked meals to your diet.

Evaluate Cultural or Culinary Preferences: Consider any influences on your food selections from a cultural or culinary standpoint. To guarantee diversity and delight, include your favorite foods or cuisines in your meal plan.

Track Eating Patterns: To spot trends and habits, keep a food journal or monitor your eating habits for a week. Make any necessary modifications to your meal plan based on this information to suit your lifestyle and nutritional requirements.

You can adjust your meal planning strategy to meet your specific demands and objectives by evaluating your own requirements and preferences. This guarantees that your meal planning will be useful, pleasurable, and long-lasting.

Putting a Meal Planning System in Place

Putting up a meal planning system entails creating a structure and schedule for effectively organizing, sourcing, and cooking meals. The following is a detailed guide to assist you in creating a meal planning system:

Select Your Planning Method: Choose the meal planning strategy that best suits your needs. This might involve utilizing a digital app or spreadsheet, a physical planner or notebook, or even just a plain whiteboard or blackboard in your kitchen.

Choose a Planning Interval: Choose the frequency at which you will schedule meals. While some prefer to plan every week, others prefer to do it every two weeks or every month.

Select a planned period that works with your buying habits and schedule.

Choose a Planning Day: Every week, set aside a particular day to plan your meals. You can choose any day that works for you to do this, even over the weekend. Set out specific time in your calendar to devote yourself entirely to meal planning.

Make a Meal Planning Template: Make a meal planning template with sections for breakfast, lunch, supper, and snacks, with room for each day of the week. You can use this template to help you organize your weekly meal plan.

Gather Recipes: To include in your meal plan, gather recipes from websites, cookbooks, or family favorites. Select meals based on your time limits, cooking abilities, and nutritional preferences.

Plan Your Meals: Make a list of the meals you will eat during the next week using the form provided. Take into account elements like ingredient availability, time limits, and dietary restrictions. To make your meal plan interesting, try to include some variation.

Make a Shopping List: Using your weekly menu as a guide, make a thorough list of all the ingredients you'll need to buy. To make your shopping trip more efficient, divide the list into categories like produce, dairy, proteins, and pantry necessities.

Purchase Ingredients: Make time to use your prepared shopping list to go grocery shopping, either in-person or online. To prevent impulsive purchases and stick to your spending limit, stick to your list.

Prepare items: To make meal preparation during the week easier, spend some time preparing items after your supermarket shopping. This can entail pre-cooking grains, marinating proteins, and cleaning and slicing veggies.

Store and Organize Ingredients: To improve the efficiency of meal preparation, store ingredients in an organized way. Perishable goods should be kept out of sight and easily accessible. Ingredients should be kept organized and fresh using storage containers.

Observe Your food Plan: Make sure you prepare meals in accordance with your schedule by consulting your food plan over the week. To expedite cooking and save time, use foods you've prepped ahead of time and leftovers.

Assess and Make Adjustments: At the conclusion of every week, assess the success of your meal plan and make any necessary adjustments. Consider what went well and what may be done better, then adjust your meal planning approach as needed.

These guidelines will help you create a meal planning system that works for you and makes it easier for you to organize, buy for, and cook meals for your family. Meal planning can become an effective tool for reducing stress, wasted time, and expenses in the kitchen with regular practice and consistency.

Finding Inspiration for Recipes

A crucial component of meal planning is gathering recipe ideas, which can serve as a source of creativity for preparing meals that are varied, savory, and well-balanced. Here are a few methods to help you get inspired by recipes when creating your meal plan:

Cookbooks: Look through a range of cookbooks to get ideas. Seek out cookbooks that highlight your favorite cooking method, diet, or cuisine. To assist you in getting started with meal planning, a lot of cookbooks also contain weekly menus or meal plans.

Online Recipe Websites: For a variety of recipe ideas, peruse well-known recipe websites and food blogs. Large recipe collections are available on websites such as Epicurious, Food Network, and Allrecipes. These collections can be searched by ingredients, cuisine, dietary restrictions, and other criteria.

Social media: Use Facebook, Instagram, Pinterest, and other social media sites to follow chefs, food bloggers, and cooking lovers. Your meal plan may be inspired by the scrumptious images and dish suggestions that frequently appear in social media feeds.

Food publications: For seasonal recipe collections, cooking advice, and meal planning recommendations, subscribe to food publications or visit their websites. There are lots of recipes in magazines like Bon Appétit, Cooking Light, and Taste of Home that are good for meal planning.

Meal Planning applications: Make use of meal planning applications that provide you with meal plans and recipe recommendations based on your cooking habits and dietary preferences. You can explore recipes, plan meals, and make shopping lists all in one location with apps like Mealime, Plan to Eat, and Paprika.

YouTube Channels: For step-by-step directions and visual inspiration, watch culinary lessons and recipe videos on YouTube. Meal prep ideas, batch cooking advice, and recipe roundups ideal for meal planning can be found on a lot of cooking channels.

Pinterest Boards: Use Pinterest to find inspiration for recipes by looking for particular ingredients, culinary styles, or dietary requirements. To make meal planning easier, make boards and bookmark your favorite recipes and meal ideas.

Cooking Classes or Workshops: To pick up new skills and get recipe ideas, sign up for cooking classes or workshops in your area or online. A lot of cooking lessons concentrate on certain cuisines or cooking techniques, which might serve as an inspiration for your meal planning.

Family and Friends: Don't forget to take advantage of their gastronomic expertise. Seek advice on recipes or discuss meal ideas with people who appreciate preparing and cooking.

Modify Pre-Existing Recipes: Adapt your favorite foods and recipes to suit your meal plan by drawing inspiration from them. To make interesting and novel meals, try experimenting with different cooking techniques, substituting ingredients, and adjusting portion sizes.

You can find a plethora of inspiration for your meal planning routine by looking through these sources of dish ideas. Try a variety of flavors, cooking methods, and cuisines to keep your menu interesting, tasty, and up to date.

Making a Weekly Schedule for Meals

Making a weekly meal schedule is a useful tool for organizing your meals ahead of time and guaranteeing that you eat a healthy, diverse diet all week long. This is how to make a weekly food planner:

Choose Your Planning Format: Make a decision regarding the layout of your meal schedule. A physical planner, an electronic calendar, a spreadsheet, or even a plain notebook or whiteboard can be used.

Select the Days of the Week: Choose the days of the week for which you will schedule your meals. Meal plans typically span seven days, but you can modify them to fit your preferences and timetable.

Think About Meal Categories: Set aside time for breakfast, lunch, supper, and snacks on each day of the week. This makes it easier to make sure you have plans for all of your meals and snacks during the day.

First, focus on the major events of the week. Take into account any unique occasions, activities, or commitments. Consider things like time limits or dietary requirements while planning meals for these occasions.

Include Variety: Throughout the week, try to incorporate a range of cuisines, cooking techniques, and ingredients into your meal plan. This helps avoid mealtime monotony and keeps meals exciting.

Balanced Nutritional Needs: Make sure that the proteins, carbs, fats, vitamins, and minerals in your meal plan are all in their proper proportions.

Throughout your meals, include a range of fruits, vegetables, nutritious grains, and lean proteins.

Use Theme Nights: To make meal planning easier, think about adding theme nights to your calendar. Set up Mondays, for instance, for spaghetti night, Tuesdays for tacos, Wednesdays for stir fries, and so on.

Consider Leftovers: When planning your meals, make sure to include leftovers by purposefully preparing additional portions that may be eaten as meals at a later time during the week. This minimizes food waste and lessens the need for additional meal preparation.

Check Your Inventory: To determine what products you already have on hand, go through your pantry, refrigerator, and freezer before finalizing your meal plan. Create menus that include these items to cut down on grocery shopping and food waste.

Make a Meal Plan: Write down specific dinner suggestions for each day of the week in your meal calendar. Add all of your planned meals, including breakfast, lunch, supper, and snacks. Don't forget to include any drinks or desserts.

Think About Prep and Cooking Times: When organizing your schedule, don't forget to factor in the amount of time needed to prepare and cook each meal. When you're pressed for time, opt for easier recipes; on other days, conserve your energy for more complex ones.

Be Adaptable: Keep in mind that your meal planner is only a suggestion, not a set timetable. Be adaptable and prepared to modify your strategy as necessary in response to shifts in your preferences, availability of ingredients, or schedule.

These instructions will help you make a weekly meal plan that will keep you organized, ensure that your meals are well-balanced, and reduce stress and time spent in the kitchen. To make sure your meal plan still suits your needs and preferences, review and adjust it on a regular basis.

Creating a Shopping List

Making a grocery list is an essential part of meal planning since it helps you avoid impulsive buys and food waste by making sure you have everything you need for the meals you have planned. To create a grocery list for your meal planning, follow these steps:

Examine Your Meal Plan: To begin, go over your weekly meal plan or schedule. Make a list of every recipe and meal you have scheduled for the next week, including snacks and dinner and breakfast.

Examine Your Fridge, Pantry, and Freezer: List all of the ingredients you currently have on hand. See if you have anything in your pantry, refrigerator, or freezer that you'll need for the meals you have planned. Any ingredients you need to refill should be noted.

Sort Your List: To make grocery shopping more effective, separate your list into several categories. Produce, dairy, proteins, cereals, canned goods, spices, and other random things are common categories.

List Particular Ingredients: Provide as much information as you can on each ingredient that will be used in the meals you have planned. In order to make sure you get the right amount of each item, including dimensions and quantities.

Think About Meal Prep Ingredients: Include these products on your grocery list if you intend to prepare ingredients ahead of time, such as by washing and cutting vegetables or marinating proteins.

Add Staples and Essentials: Remember to include basic foods and necessities that you frequently use, such bread, milk, eggs, cooking oil, and spices, in addition to the ingredients for the meals you have planned.

Look for Sales and Discounts: Look through online or sales flyer advertisements to find deals on the things you need. To reduce the amount you spend on groceries, take advantage of bargains and promotions.

Be Aware of Quantity: Make sure your list reflects the amounts of each component you'll need for your meals. Steer clear of overspending on perishables to reduce food waste.

Consider Seasonality: In season produce is typically fresher and more reasonably priced, so choose for fruits and veggies wherever possible. Additionally, seasonal produce is more likely to be discounted, saving you money.

Make a Plan for Breakfast and Snacks: Don't forget to add breakfast and snack ingredients to your grocery list. Think of simple and convenient options such as fruit, nuts, yogurt, cereal, and snack bars.

Double-Check Your List: To make sure you haven't forgotten any ingredients, compare your final grocery list to your meal plan. As needed, make any required alterations or additions.

Keep to Your List: Try your best to avoid making impulsive purchases when you go food shopping by sticking to your list. Throughout your shopping journey, consult your list to maintain concentration and direction.

These steps will help you make a thorough grocery list that will guarantee you have everything you need for the meals you have planned, saving you money, time, and headaches when you go shopping.

Astute Purchasing Techniques

Using smart shopping techniques can help you plan meals more efficiently, save time and money, and reduce food waste. The following are some wise purchasing tactics to think about:

Make a Detailed Shopping List: Using your meal plan and inventory as a guide, make a thorough shopping list before you go shopping. Make a list of all the ingredients you'll need for the meals you have planned, along with any necessities or staples.

Plan Your Shopping Trip: To cut down on wait times and distractions, go shopping at a time when the store is less crowded. To optimize savings, bring reusable shopping bags and any required discount cards or coupons.

Keep to Your Budget: Prior to your food shop, decide on a spending limit and follow it. Steer clear of impulsive buys and concentrate on purchasing just the things on your list. To assist you in staying within your budget, think about using cash or an app for food shopping.

Shop the Periphery: Begin your shopping expedition by circling the store's perimeter, which is usually home to the fresh produce, dairy, meat, and seafood departments. The healthiest, least processed foods can be found in these places.

Buy in Bulk for Staples: To save money over time, think about buying staples like grains, legumes, nuts, and spices in large quantities. For more affordable solutions, look for larger package sizes or bulk bins.

Examine Prices and Unit Costs: To be sure you're receiving the greatest deal possible, compare the prices and unit costs of comparable items. On things you frequently use, keep an eye out for promotions, discounts, and deals.

Select Seasonal Produce: Because they are generally more inexpensive, fresher, and more tasty, seasonal fruits and vegetables are the better choice. Additionally, seasonal produce is more likely to be discounted, saving you money.

Verify Expiration Dates: Prior to making a purchase, always verify the expiration dates and quality of perishable goods. To reduce food waste, select products with the greatest shelf life possible.

Think About Store Brands: Check for cost savings by comparing name brands and store brands' costs. Store brands frequently provide same quality for less money.

Limit Processed Foods: Because processed and convenience foods are typically more expensive and less nutrient-dense, try to avoid buying them. To cut costs and encourage better eating habits, concentrate on full, unadulterated meals and ingredients.

Be Versatile with Brands: If you want to save money, don't be afraid to try generic or alternative brands for some products. It's possible that you can pay less for something of comparable quality.

Avoid Shopping When Hungry: Buying on the spur of the moment and going over budget are risks associated with grocery shopping. Have a lunch or snack before you go shopping to help you make more sensible and cost-effective decisions.

You can maximize your meal planning efforts and grocery shopping experience by putting these clever shopping techniques into practice. You'll save time and money doing it too.

Getting Ready for Meal Prep

Meal prep must be done in advance to guarantee a seamless and effective cooking experience. The following is how to prepare for meal prep:

Plan Your Meals: To begin, arrange your meals for the upcoming week. Choose the meals you'll be cooking, keeping in mind your availability of ingredients, dietary restrictions, and schedule.

Recipe Selection: Opt for recipes that work well for meal preparation and are simple to portion out and store. Seek for dishes that are easy to prepare in big quantities, healthy, and straightforward.

Make a Shopping List: Using the recipes you've selected, make a thorough list of all the ingredients you'll need. Make a list of all the ingredients you currently have and check your pantry and refrigerator to determine what is missing.

Stock Up on Meal Prep Containers: To preserve your cooked meals, get a set of reusable meal prep containers in different sizes. For optimal versatility, use freezer-safe, dishwasher-safe, and microwave-safe containers.

Assemble Kitchen Utensils and Tools: Before beginning any meal preparation, make sure you have all the cooking utensils, pots, pans, mixing bowls, knives, and cutting boards you'll need. Think about purchasing time-saving appliances such as a food processor, slow cooker, or instant pot.

Plan Meal Prep Time: Allocate a specific period of time in your calendar for meal preparation. Every week, pick one or two days when you have the most time to cook and prepare meals ahead of time.

Select a Meal Prep Area: Set aside a section of your kitchen where you can prepare meals with plenty of counter space and easy access to the supplies you'll need. Keep your desk clean, organized, and free of clutter to improve efficiency.

Examine Recipes and Instructions: Get acquainted with the recipes you'll be making and go over any guidelines or tips for cooking. Cooking can be sped up by preparing materials ahead of time, such as cutting and cleaning veggies or marinating meats.

Batch Cooking: To save time and effort, think about batch cooking some of your meal's ingredients, such as grains, proteins, or sauces. Make big batches of these and divide them into meal prep containers so they're simple to assemble later.

Label Containers: To help you remember what's inside and when it was created, label meal prep containers with the name of the dish and the date it was prepared. Throughout the week, this makes it simpler to retrieve meals from the freezer or refrigerator.

Make sure your kitchen is spotless and well-organized before beginning to prepare meals. To make a kitchen space that is ideal for cooking, clean the dishes, dust the surfaces, and remove any clutter.

Keep Yourself Hydrated and Energized: Throughout the meal prep process, maintain your energy levels by keeping a water bottle close at hand and indulging in nutritious snacks like yogurt, nuts, or fruit. You may avoid being fatigued and maintain attention by taking brief breaks to rest and replenish your energy.

You can speed up the cooking process, save time, and position yourself for success throughout the week by planning ahead for meal prep. Meal prep becomes a practical and effective way to regularly enjoy tasty, homemade meals with the right preparation and organization.

Following through with your weekly meal plan, which includes grocery shopping, meal preparation, and meal storage, is known as "execution." Here's how to successfully carry out your meal plan:

Grocery Shopping: Prepare your shopping list in advance and head out to the grocery store. In order to prevent impulsive purchases and keep inside your budget, try your best to adhere to your list. To reduce wait times and distractions, think about scheduling your shopping for a time when the store is less crowded.

Meal Prep: Schedule specific time to prepare your meals ahead of time. You can decide to meal prep in batches throughout the week or all at once, depending on your preferences and schedule. To wash, chop, cook, and portion out ingredients for each meal, go to your recipes and meal plan.

Cooking: To achieve the greatest results, meticulously follow the recipes and directions when it comes time to cook your meals. When cooking, try to cook in batches to reduce cleanup time and save time. To expedite the cooking process, think about utilizing time-saving gadgets like sheet pans, quick pots, or slow cookers.

After your meals are prepared, divide them into portions and store them in meal prep containers. For ease of identification, write the dish's name and preparation date on the label of each container. Meals should be kept chilled or frozen based on their shelf life and reheating guidelines.

Reheating and Serving: Just follow the directions to reheat your premade meals in the oven, stovetop, or microwave when it's time to eat.

CHAPTER THREE

Enjoy your own dishes and add extra toppings or decorations as preferred to your meals.

Remain Adaptable: Adjust your meal plan as necessary to accommodate shifts in your preferences, schedule, or the availability of ingredients. Don't be afraid to make changes as needed, such as switching out a meal or adjusting portion amounts.

Track Food Inventory: Throughout the week, keep an eye on your food supply to make sure you have enough food for until your next scheduled grocery shop. If necessary, modify your meal plan or prepare extra meals to prevent running out of food.

Reduce Food Waste: Use perishable items before they go bad and repurpose leftovers into new meals to help reduce food waste. Use leftovers in inventive ways by adding them to stir-fries, salads, and sandwiches.

Clean Up: After preparing meals and cooking activities, don't forget to tidy up your kitchen. To keep your workspace tidy and orderly, wash dishes, clean surfaces, and store unused components appropriately.

Evaluate and Modify: At the conclusion of the week, give yourself some time to consider how your food plan performed. Think on what went well and what could be done better for your next meal planning endeavors. Make any future necessary adjustments to your food plan based on this feedback.

These guidelines will help you carry out your meal plan efficiently and reap the rewards of having delectable, handmade meals available all week long. Meal prep becomes a practical and effective strategy to consistently eat well-balanced meals with the right preparation and organization.

Assessing and Modifying the Meal Schedule

To make sure the meal plan stays effective and suits your needs and preferences, it is essential to evaluate and make adjustments to it. The following are some ways to assess and modify your food plan:

Think Back on the Week: Give yourself some time to consider how your weekly food plan performed. Think on things like the variety of meals, how simple they were to prepare, how satisfying they were to taste, whether you stuck to your budget, and if you had enough food for the entire week.

Evaluate Input: Collect input from relatives or other diners you eat with. Find out what they thought of the meals, what they enjoyed and didn't like, and if they have any advice for how to prepare meals going forward.

Evaluate Food Inventory: Look over your food inventory to determine whether you have any meals or ingredients left over that need to be consumed. To reduce food waste, use these things as ideas for new meals or as a starting point for meal planning in the future.

Think About Lifestyle Changes: If your schedule, way of life, or dietary preferences change, it may have an impact on how often you need to arrange your meals. Make the necessary adjustments to your food plan to reflect these developments and make sure it stays feasible and realistic.

Identify Challenges: List any difficulties or roadblocks you had this week, such as limited time, trouble locating specific ingredients, or unsuccessful attempts at recipes. When you plan meals in the future, come up with some alternatives or answers to these problems.

Make Modifications: Adapt your meal plan as necessary in light of your reflections and input. This may include experimenting with different recipes, adding diversity to your meals, modifying portion sizes, or altering your habits for grocery shopping and cooking.

Establish Goals: Whether it's to make more home-cooked meals, include more veggies in your diet, or stay inside a certain budget, set precise goals for your future meal planning. Use these objectives as a reference to help you plan your meals.

Think forward: Arrange your meals for the coming week by looking forward. Create a new meal plan that tackles any problems or opportunities for improvement using the knowledge you've gained from assessing your current one.

Remain adaptive: When it comes to meal preparation, never forget to remain flexible and adaptive. It's acceptable to adjust your strategy as necessary to account for unforeseen events or circumstances because life can be unpredictable.

Monitor Your Progress: As you go with your meal planning endeavor, keep a record of your advancements and successes. Celebrate your victories and take lessons from failures to keep getting better at food planning.

You can make sure that your meal plan stays efficient, fun, and in line with your preferences and goals by reviewing and modifying it on a frequent basis. Meal planning may help you enjoy tasty and nourishing meals while saving money, time, and stress in the kitchen with regular practice and consistency.

CONCLUSION

To sum up, establishing a meal plan is an effective and proactive way to control how much food you eat, save time and money, and encourage healthier eating practices. You can reap many advantages by putting into practice a methodical meal planning procedure, including:

Time Savings: By streamlining your meal preparation process and saving you significant time during hectic weekdays, meal planning removes the need for impromptu food decisions.

Financial Savings: You may prevent impulsive purchases, cut down on food waste, and make more cost-effective decisions by making a shopping list based on your meal plan and adhering to it. This will help you save money on groceries.

Better Eating Habits: By controlling portion sizes, incorporating a range of nutrient-dense foods into your diet, and making deliberate food choices, meal planning helps you maintain a balanced and healthful eating schedule.

Decreased Stress: Being aware of the meals you'll be having each week helps reduce the anxiety and stress that comes with mealtimes, enabling you to approach preparing and eating with poise and readiness.

Enhanced Variety: Meal planning gives you the chance to try out new recipes, cuisines, and ingredients, so your meals are more fascinating, fun, and diverse.

Environmental Benefits: You may lessen your influence on the environment and promote a more sustainable lifestyle by minimizing food waste via thoughtful meal planning and ingredient management.

In order to begin meal planning successfully, you must first evaluate your own needs, preferences, and goals. Then, you must make a shopping list and meal plan, then carry out your plan by cooking meals ahead of time. To guarantee your meal plan's continuous success, review it frequently and make any adjustments based on feedback and experiences.

Making meal planning a regular part of your routine will help you take charge of your eating choices, streamline the preparation process, and reap the many advantages of conscious and well-organized eating habits. Meal planning can be a useful tool for reaching your financial, lifestyle, and health objectives with regular practice.

THE END